Jimmy Joe Jam Has Sickle Cell Disease

by

Dr. Dorcas T. Saunders

ISBN 13: 978=1517342319
ISBN-10: 1517342317

DEDICATION

This book is dedicated to my grand children:

Jamal, Leah, Matthew, Fred, Isaac, Isaiah, Connie and Carzzett's son as well as my great-grand children:

Xavier, Chase & Caleb

And my husband Israel Shannon Saunders

CONTENTS

ACKNOWLEDGMENTS

First and foremost I'd like to thank my highest
power, God, who placed the gifting in me
in the first place and to say it is truly making
way for me. I'd also like to acknowledge
the following people in my life that love
children just like I do. My daughter
Tonya whose quiver is full. There's my
husband, Israel, who encourages me
and my dad, Mr. Melvin, God rest
his soul, and dog Co-co. There are
many others that I didn't mention
because if I did this would be a
book of acknowledgements.

From the Author

When reading this book to your children
(ages pre-k and up) I suggest that you
allow the child(ren) to look at the
words as you point to them. Repeat
these reading sessions with this book
several times a week. After each session
discuss Jimmy Joe Jam's experience.

Jimmy Joe Jam Has Sickle Cell Disease

Jimmy Joe Jam is a little boy that has SCD.

One day while playing with his friends,

He fell to his knees.

His friends thought he was playing a game,

They thought it was a joke.

Jimmy Joe Jam was not playing,

He had just had a stroke.

He was only 9 years old

and it took him for a loop;

a stroke at 9, that was unheard of,

at least not in his SCD group.

When he got to the hospital

And he was examined,

It was confirmed...a stroke he did have.

He couldn't walk, he couldn't talk

But, his life was saved.

Early detection of the symptoms

kept him alive,

And the medication that he was given

helped him survive.

When he got to the hospital and he was examined

The doctor told his mom;

She looked at the doctor with a puzzled expression

And she out of shock said, "WHAT!"

The information was too much and

She thought, "But he's only 9."

The doctor said, "Look at it this way,

He will recover with time.

But one thing we know in cases like this

We have to be alert;

If he had one stroke there may be another,

Regardless of how we work."

But in Jimmy's mom's mind

She heard a voice say, "whose

Report will you believe?"

She knew right then her God

Had spoken and then her stress

Was relieved.

She began praying and Jimmy got

Better even though he still had SCD.

Then a miracle occurred

There was a procedure

That could take away SCD.

But there was a chance

It would not work,

But with God that

They needed a donor

Of bone marrow you know

As the prayers were

steady going up,

more blessings were coming

and Jimmy's family was hopeful

as God was steadily filling their cup.

A relative was needed to make

It a better chance to work,

Then up stepped his sister to

Volunteer to donate, man

What a brave little girl.

The procedure was a success,

Jimmy's family was glad and

Praised God for what He had done;

Their prayers were heard

And between the Lord and His Word

This battle had been won.

ABOUT THE AUTHOR

Dorcas Saunders lives in Chapel Hill, North Carolina (home
 of the Tar Heels), with her husband Israel Shannon Saunder.
 She has three children eight grandchildren and three
great grand children. She has an outreach ministry,
 (Dorcas Saunders Ministries), through which she
 gives food away in cooperation with the North Carolina
Food Bank of Durham, North Carolina.
She writes poetry regularly. Dorcas loves writing poetry
 for and about children. In the following pages you
 will find a couple of her poems. Enjoy!

I Think I'll...

I think I'll.....
Ask my mommy if I can go to my friend Inky's house,
His mom just brought him a neat white mouse;
It doesn't have a name quite yet,
Man! I wish I had my very own pet.

My cousin Soupy has a cat,
She gave her cat a ball of yarn to bat:
Her cat's name is Tinky-Ray,
That's a funny name for me to say.

I Think I'll....
Wait for dad to come home,
His job keeps him away for so long;
I miss my dad and he works so hard,

Running his brother's lumber yard.

I like to see the big trucks roll,
Some carry logs that look like light poles;
I like to hear the big saw buzz,
The dust on the floor looks like wood fuzz.

With all this thinking I'm getting tired,
I think I'll eat some chocolate and just get
Wired....!

How Come?

How come when the sun comes up it is yellow;
 and when it goes down it is orange and red;
How come bears sleep all winter on the floor of a cave,
Whatever happened to their warm cozy bed?

How come grandpa's ears have hair growing out,
And when we talk about them it makes him pout;
How come when we make his suspenders pop,
He turns around and gives our bottom a whop?

How come tree leaves are green in summer,
And in winter they are brown;
Why are squirrels all skinny in winter,
And in summer they are fat and round?

How come mommy turned on the faucet,
And water flew everywhere?
Daddy fixed it just last night,
When he said the pipe had a tear.

And how come cats have kittens and
Chickens all lay eggs,
And dogs have puppies in the closet
And not on the bed?

CHILDREN

Children are a blessing from the Lord,
The Bible tells me so;
Blessed is he that has his quiver full,
These words do make me glow.

Rearing them gives you youth,
Botoks you most definitely won't need;

During the day they'll run you around,
At night you'll be on your knees.

As you watch your babies grow
Into toddlers,

The joy of watching them waddle around,
I cannot put into words.

Then there comes those teenage years
Of which you will shed many tears,
Remember the Lord and His Word,
They both will disperse all your fears.

Finally remember to raise up children
In the Way they should go,
Put nothing but Life in them;
The Word is the Way
 though they may Go astray
 and their paths might look kind of dim.

CHILDREN
(continued)

When they become adults
And have children of their own,
You'll think 'My how they've grown',
It was just yesterday,
When they would run and play,
Now they have Children of their own.

Jimmy Joe Jam Has Sickle Cell Disease

Epilogue to the parents

As we walk through life we have situations that
we are confronted with on a daily basis. How
we go through the motions of dealing with these
situations determines whether we repeat
these situations or not. Do we learn from them
or do we go through them over and over and
over again until we do? Patience is needed in
the event we do continually go through these
situations. We need to have patience with others
as well as patience with ourselves. It is written, "Let
patience have her perfect work", James 1:4 King James
Version of the Bible and it also states that, "Tribulation
worketh patience", Romans 5:3 KJV of the Bible.
Jimmy had to exercise patience as he went through
the episodes with his the sickle cell disease, in
pursuit of relief from it. His mother didn't give
up or let go of her faith in God, even after the
doctors gave her a report that didn't
look good. She just continued to walk by faith
and not by sight. God loves us in that we trust
Him in that way. We sometimes go off on a tangent
or on another path. We should just continue to

The Reveal

The revelation is that I wrote this book based on the experiences of my husband and his family. My husband had Sickle Cell Anemia at birth but was not diagnosed till he was 6 months old. His bone marrow transplant happened when he was 14 years old. During the time he was battling Sickle Cell Anemia he had a stroke at the age of 10 years old. I thank God for the people and the prayers that were existent in his life at that time. At the age of 35 years old he is still Sickle Cell anemia free. There are still issues he has to deal with in his body. The disease caused permanent damage to his eyes and there are problems with his hearing. Miracles still happen today and we are believing God all the way.

NOTES:

THE BEGINNING ☺

.

www.ingramcontent.com/pod-product-compliance
Lightning Source LLC
Chambersburg PA
CBHW070801180526
45168CB00004B/1701